Alzheimer's Book

Diagnosis, Treatment, and Risk Reduction Strategies

There is a tsunami coming. Not a tsunami from the sea, but a healthcare tsunami of Alzheimer's patients. For every patient officially diagnosed with Alzheimer's, many more are living with this condition undiagnosed.

Alzheimer's disease is currently the 6th leading cause of death in the United States. It is projected to become the 4th leading cause of death by year 2030.

It is common to hear about people who have survived heart attacks, strokes, and cancer – however there are no survivors of Alzheimer's disease.

Some of the chapters in this book talk about:

- The upcoming epidemic
- Cognitive Symptoms
- 3 Buckets of Alzheimer's Causes
- 6 Pillars of Risk Reduction

If Alzheimer's disease concerns you pick up a copy of this powerful book today.

Your Amazing Itty Bitty® Alzheimer's Book

Diagnosis, Treatment, and Risk Reduction Strategies

Dung Trinh, MD

Published by Itty Bitty® Publishing
A subsidiary of S & P Productions, Inc.

Copyright © 2018 Dung Trinh, MD

Printed in the United States of America

Itty Bitty Publishing
311 Main Street, Suite D
El Segundo, CA 90245
(310) 640-8885

ISBN: 978-1-950326-00-6

Dedication Page

This book is dedicated to the many patients and their families I have treated over the years who have suffered from Alzheimer's disease. In the past we physicians have dreaded making this diagnosis - as it implies a prognosis that is pointed in one direction without hope.

But hope is coming. Our clinical trials are shedding more light to this condition as we make incremental progress towards slowing down and hopefully one day preventing this dreaded disease.

While we wait for medications in the clinical research pipeline to come to fruition, there is much that we can still do. Lifestyle activities such as appropriate diet and nutrition to getting adequate sleep and socializing with our family and friends may play a protective role in brain health.

Lowering your risk for Alzheimer's can start today. My hope is that this small Itty Bitty book may motivate many to make lifestyle changes that will affect their brain health for years to come.

Stop by our Itty Bitty® website Directory to find to interesting information about Alzheimer's Disease.

www.IttyBittyPublishing.com

Or visit Dr Dung Trinh at:

HealthyBrainClub.com

Table of Contents

Step 1
Alzheimer's: An
Upcoming Epidemic

There is a tsunami coming. Not a tsunami from the sea, but a healthcare tsunami of Alzheimer's patients. For every patient officially diagnosed with Alzheimer's, many more are living with this condition undiagnosed.

1. Alzheimer's disease is currently the 6th leading cause of death in the United States. It is projected to become the 4th leading cause of death by year 2030.
2. More than five million Americans are estimated to have Alzheimer's in the United States. This number is expected to triple by year 2050.
3. While death rates from heart attacks, strokes, and cancer have been decreasing due to advancing treatments and prevention – the number of deaths from Alzheimer's have increased over 100% in the last 10 years.
4. This disease costs the nation over $200 billion in 2017. That rate is expected to rise to $1.2 trillion by the year 2050.
5. It is common to hear about people who have survived heart attacks, strokes, and cancer – however there are no survivors of Alzheimer's disease.

Questions to Think About

- Are you blaming your memory loss problems on "old age"?
- Are you getting a yearly Brain Health Exam that includes a memory test to screen for early dementia?
- Do you know someone who is struggling and may need help with their memory loss?

Are you Prepared for the Future?

- Do you have a Will and/or Living Trust set up?
- Do you have an Advance Directive Form in place for Medical Decision making and Financial Decision making?
- Do you have a Physician Order for Life Sustaining Treatment (POLST) Form in place?
- Have you thought about potential Long Term Care needs such as nursing home and assisted living?

Step 2
Diagnosis: Cognitive Symptoms

We all forget. Forgetfulness can occur at any age.

Your brain stores memory like a file cabinet in which memories are stored in chronological order. With Alzheimer's disease, memories are destroyed beginning with the most recent ones and ending with the oldest. Here's how to differentiate between harmless and dangerous memory loss.

Normal Memory Loss (Harmless)

1. Intermittent
2. Non progressive
3. Random

Abnormal Memory Loss

1. Progressively worsens over time
2. Frequent forgetfulness
3. Initial short term memory loss
4. Eventual long term memory loss.

Do You Have Any of These Symptoms?

- Confusion with Time or Places
- Problems with Speaking or Writing
- Memory Loss that Disrupts Daily Life
- Difficulty Completing Familiar Tasks
- Decreased or Poor Judgment
- Challenges in Planning or Solving Problems
- Misplacing Things and Losing the Ability to Retrace Steps
- Withdrawal from Work or Social Activities

If you have one or more of these symptoms you should consider consulting your doctor to discuss these concerns.

Step 3
Diagnosis:
Scanning an Alzheimer's Brain

A Normal Brain:

1. A healthy brain has 100,000,000,000 brain cells (neurons).
2. In a healthy brain, one brain cell will speak to the next brain cell, which will speak to the next brain cell and so on.
3. Each memory can be viewed as a specific pattern of connection between brain cells to brain cells.

The Alzheimer's Brain:

1. Amyloid beta plaques and Tau "tangles" build up excessively in the brain.
4. The plaques interrupt communication pathways between brain cells.
4. Brain cells are no longer able to communicate with each other and eventually die over time.
5. The brain shrinks in size over time.
6. Memory loss occurs as a result of disrupted brain cell communication and brain cell death.

Scans to Detect Alzheimer's

Alzheimer's MRI Brain Scan:

- In early stages of Alzheimer's, an MRI of the brain may appear normal.
- The volume of the brain decreases over time.
- The temporal and parietal lobes decrease in size. The hippocampus is usually affected first.

Amyloid PET Brain Scan:

- Amyloid tracer will tag amyloid beta plaque in the brain and highlight these plaque on the scan. This scan is FDA approved.

Tau PET Brain Scan:

- Tau tracer designed to detect Tau tangles on a PET scan – available only under a clinical research setting. Tau PET brain scan is not FDA approved as of this writing.

Step 4
Current Medication Options

In the brain, neurons communicate with one another at "synapses", where small chemicals called neurotransmitters transmit information from one neuron to another.

In Alzheimer's disease, amyloid beta plaque disrupt the communication network between brain cell to brain cell, leading to neuron damage and death.

There are currently four FDA approved Alzheimer's medications designed to support the brain communication process.

1. Donezepil (Aricept) - approved 1996
2. Rivastigmine (Exelon) - approved 2000
3. Galantamine (Razadyne) - approved 2001
4. Memantine (Namenda) - approved 2003

Some Thoughts About the Current FDA Approved Medications:

- These medications can temporarily slow the worsening of symptoms.
- These medications do not slow down the progression of Alzheimer's disease.
- These medications do not stop the build up of amyloid beta plaque or tau tangles over time.
- The last unique FDA approved medication for Alzheimer's disease was developed over 15 years ago.
- Between 2002 and 2012, over 400 clinical trials were conducted on Alzheimer's disease with a 99.6% failure rate.
- Since the last FDA approved medication in 2003, there has been no success in finding a new medication to slow down or prevent Alzheimer's disease.

Step 5
Three Buckets of Alzheimer's Causes
1. Circulation

Any condition that causes poor circulation to the body will increase the risk for having Alzheimer's disease.

Statistics show that out of every 10 patients with Alzheimer's:

1. Eight have hypertension (high blood pressure).
2. Four have diabetes.
3. Three have heart disease.
4. Many have high cholesterol, obesity, and poor physical fitness.

Any condition that is a risk factor for heart disease is also a risk factor for Alzheimer's.

Circulation Risk Factors for Alzheimer's Disease

- Diabetics and those with high cholesterol have double the risk of Alzheimer's compared to those without these conditions.
- High blood pressure, Diabetes, cardiac disease – If these conditions are under control with lifestyle and medications then risk factors for Alzheimer's is reduced as well.
- To reduce Alzheimer's risk, those with risk of heart disease need to modify their lifestyle since both conditions share the same risk factors.
- Sleep apnea not treated is a risk factor due to the lack of adequate oxygenation to the brain.
- Any lifestyle activities that improve circulation will also lower risk for Alzheimer's.

Step 6
Three Buckets of Alzheimer's Causes
2. Inflammation

Inflammation conditions can affect any organ system of our body. When inflammation becomes chronic, it increases risk of Alzheimer's.

Chronic organ system inflammation and associated pathologic diagnosis:

1. Skin – eczema, dermatitis, psoriasis, etc.
2. Lungs – allergic asthma.
3. GI tract – crohn's disease, ulcerative colitis, celiac disease.
4. Joints – rheumatoid arthritis, psoriatic arthritis.
5. Kidney – glomerulonephritis.
6. Brain – Alzheimer's disease (high number of inflammatory cells found in brains of Alzheimer's patients at autopsies).

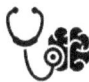

Inflammation and Alzheimer's Disease

Inflammation does not come only from chronic medical conditions. Inflammation can also come from food sources and environmental exposure.

Pro-inflammatory foods:

- Red Meat
- Margarine and all other hydrogenated fats and oils
- Cheese
- Sugar (Pastries, cookies, candy, etc)
- Fried Food
- Fast Food

Advanced glycation end-product (AGE):

- AGEs are proteins that are "glycated" (attached sugar molecule) which promotes "oxidative stress" and inflammation.
- High blood sugar in diabetes promote AGE formation due to increase availability of glucose (sugar).
- AGEs play a significant role in the formation and progression of atherosclerotic lesions, poor circulation, and Alzheimer's disease.

Step 7
Three Buckets of Alzheimer's Causes
3. Toxins

Toxins can come from the air as well as food and water.

1. Research shows that those who live in areas of high pollution have a higher risk of Alzheimer's diagnosis compared to those who live in areas of low pollution.

Toxins can come from your diet as well. If you eat red meat, you are not just eating an animal. You are also eating:

1. Hormones injected into farm animals to speed up growth for faster corporate profits.
2. Antibiotics given to animals to prevent infections.
3. Anything that was fed to the cow – including parts of other cows.
4. Pesticides that may have been sprayed on grass fed to animals.

The Toxins We Live With

- When the immune system is exposed to toxins, its first impulse is to produce "Inflammation" to defend the body.
- Today's farmed foods are no longer recognizable by our immune system due to genetic modification of many vegetables and fruits.
- Chemicals and preservatives make food unrecognizable to the immune system, which defends the body by producing inflammation.
- Chemical additives in prepared foods have a similar effect. A basic rule is: if you can't pronounce an ingredient – don't eat it.

Step 8
Risk Reduction: Six Pillars

Optimizing brain function is possible without the need to take an extra pill. These "Six Pillars" of Brain Health are the result of published clinical trials.

1. Physical Exercise
2. Brain Exercise
3. Diet and Nutrition
4. Adequate Sleep
5. Social Engagement
6. Controlling medical conditions.

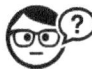

The Million Dollar Question has always been: Is Alzheimer's Preventable?

Here are some thoughts regarding this question:

- There are people around the world in other countries who live as long as Americans do without Alzheimer's on the top of their list of diagnoses.
- These people have different lifestyles, different diets and nutrition and a different culture when it comes to physical activity.
- Alzheimer's seems to affect countries that are affluent, where citizens have access to food 24/7, where red meat and sugar are more readily available and where lifestyle tends to be sedentary.
- "Modernized countries" that have technology to genetically modify food, chemically preserve and process food, and have less available organic food, seem to have a higher incidence of Alzheimer's disease.

Step 9
Physical Exercise

Physical exercise of at least 30-minutes a day has been shown to help both the heart and brain.

1. Physical exercise does not have to be stringent like running, jogging, or bicycling. A nice brisk walk of 30-minutes a day would be adequate.
2. For those who cannot exercise 30-minutes a day, consider doing 15-minutes of exercise twice a day, or 10-minutes of exercise three times a day.
3. Exercise improves blood circulation – which addresses the Circulation Bucket of Causes.
4. Exercise has been shown in clinical studies to decrease the risk of Alzheimer's diagnosis, and for those who do get diagnosed, a lifetime of good exercise habits delay the time till onset of symptoms.
5. Exercise can come in a variety of forms: Balance, Flexibility (stretching), Aerobic endurance, Strength Training.

Action Step Questions

- How much exercise are you doing each day?
- How much exercise do you need to do?
- What are the barriers to your daily exercise goal?
- What is your first step towards your goal?

Step 10
Brain Exercise

Your brain cells can still make new connections with learning at any age. When you challenge your brain to think and learn, you apply the "use it or lose it" concept – use the brain and keep it healthy, or don't use the brain and "lose it" over time. Some tips on brain exercises:

1. Choose activities that challenge your mind.
2. Learn new skills.
3. Engage multiple senses such as learning to cook a new recipe (smell, taste, sight, sound).
4. Engage your brain in different ways at the same time – socializing, fine-motor skills, learning and applying new information.

Ideas for Brain Exercises:

- Take a class - learn something challenging with a group of people.
- Teach a class – this requires you to think about how to communicate your message. You'll interact with students and engage in brain stimulating discussions.
- Plan and organize – join a club or committee that requires you to plan events, make decisions, organize information, and socialize with others.
- Try a new hobby – choose something that is challenging and requires coordination and fine motor skills (quilting, knitting, etc).
- Enhance your knowledge on a topic that interests you - sign up for classes and events at local community centers.
- Take up crossword puzzles, sudoku, chess, checkers, etc.
- Read a book, newspaper or magazine!
- Write a short book about something you are interested in or an expert in.

Step 11
Nutrition: MIND Diet (Healthy)

MIND stands for Mediterranean-DASH Intervention for Neurodegenerative Delay. This diet published in clinical research has consistently shown to reduce Alzheimer's risk.

1. Green leafy vegetables: spinach, salad greens, etc. At least six servings per week.
2. Other vegetables. At least daily.
3. Nuts: almonds, walnuts, pistachios, etc. At least five servings per week.
4. Berries: blackberry, blueberry, raspberry, etc. At least two servings per week.
5. Beans: black bean, pinto bean, refried bean. At least three servings per week.
6. Whole grain: emphasis is on "whole" which is fiber. At least three servings per day.
7. Fish: At least once a week.
8. Poultry: Chicken or turkey. At least twice a week.
9. Olive Oil: use for salads and main cooking oil.
10. Wine: 1 glass of red wine a day for those who already drink wine.

Food to Avoid (NOT Brain Healthy)

- Red Meat: less than 4 servings per week.
- Butter: less than 1-tablespoon daily.
- Margarine and all hydrogenated fats and oils should be avoided all together.
- Cheese: less than 1 serving per week.
- Pastries and sweets: less than five-servings per week.
- Fried or fast food: less than one serving per week.

In one study of the Mind Diet, the data showed that people who stuck to this diet lowered their risk of Alzheimer's disease by 54%.

Step 12
Adequate Sleep

Good Sleep is needed for good health. Here is how sleep affects the body:

1. Immune system is weakened if sleep deprived. (Sleep deprivation increases the risk of respiratory infections such as cold or flu).
2. Tissue and wound healing occurs during sleep (the body "recharges" itself).
3. Pain control improves with sleep. Lack of sleep exacerbates sensation of pain.
4. Cardiovascular health – Increase heart disease associated with lack of sleep (less than five hours at night).
5. Reaction time is impaired with poor sleep (increase risk for car accidents due to slow reaction time).
6. Balance is poor with lack of sleep (increase risk of falls).
7. Cognitive brain function is poor with lack of sleep (amyloid plaque is actively removed during sleep).

How to Improve Sleep:

- Go to bed and wake up same time each day.
- Use your bed only for sleep.
- Develop a relaxing bedtime routine.
- Avoid excessive daytime napping.
- Avoid sleep aids that may cause tolerance.
- Make your sleeping environment relaxing.

Activities to avoid 3-4 hours before bedtime:

- Moderate to vigorous exercise.
- Caffeinated drinks and food.
- Alcohol and smoking.
- Eating large meal or spicy food.
- Excessive liquid intake.

Step 13
Social Engagement

Staying socially active and maintaining relationships can help promote physical, emotional, and brain health.

Benefits of Social Engagement:

1. Reduce risk for heart problems, osteoporosis, diabetes, and arthritis due to increase in physical mobility.
2. Reduce risk for mental health issues such as depression from social isolation.
3. Increase opportunities for more physical exercise when socially engaged.
4. Protect against illness by boosting immune system.
5. May reduce risk for Alzheimer's disease.

Tips for Keeping Strong Social Engagement:

- Attend family events and enjoy the company of friends.
- Volunteer in your local community.
- Join a group focused activity you enjoy doing, such as playing bridge, drawing art, reading club, golf, or your favorite hobby.
- Try taking a class to learn something new, such as a foreign language or cooking.
- Join a gym and participate in regular group exercise classes.
- Find an organization such as a church or temple where you can stay connected and supported.
- Get involved in a movement or cause where you can share a common sense of purpose with others.
- Teaching the next generation is a great way to use your experience, interests and talents to work with others earlier in their careers.

Step 14
Control Medical Conditions

Medical Conditions Associated with Poor Brain Health:

1. Heart disease
2. Diabetes
3. High Blood Pressure
4. Obesity
5. High Cholesterol
6. Elevated Homocysteine
7. Depression
8. Low Vitamin D, B6, B12, Folate, A, C, E

Health Condition and Clinical Trial References:

A plant based (MIND) diet can improve each medical condition and as a result reduce your risk factors for Alzheimer's.

- Heart disease - Clinical Cardiology 2006; Journal of Family Practice 2014.
- Diabetes - Diabetes Care 2006; European Journal Clinical Nutrition 2013; PLoS One 2016.
- Hypertension - Nutritional Metabolic Cardiovascular Disease 2015.
- Obesity - Diabetes Care 2006; European Journal Clinical Nutrition 2013; Nutrition 2015.
- High Cholesterol - Diabetes Care 2006; European Journal Clinical Nutrition 2013.
- Homocysteine - Journal Nutrition 2000; British Journal Nutrition 2003.
- Depression - American Journal of Health Promotion 2015.
- Low Vitamin B6, folate, A, C, E - American Journal of Clinical Nutrition 2009; PLoS One 2016.

Step 15
Future Hope

We are gaining traction towards improved diagnosis and treatment through clinical research.

1. The National Institute of Aging and Alzheimer's Association has updated criteria used to define Alzheimer's disease - with a focus on objective pathophysiological findings for diagnosis.
2. As of this writing, several phase two studies have shown the ability of monoclonal antibodies to reduce beta amyloid plaque in the brain as well as slow down cognitive decline compared to control groups.
3. More light has been shed on the significance of ketosis and intermittent fasting on improving brain health - and consequently more studies are focused on this area of study.
4. Research is moving toward the direction of prevention and treatment at the earlier stages of Alzheimer's disease and pre-Alzheimer's disease.

While We Wait.

While we are waiting for the next FDA-Approved Alzheimer's medication, there are several action items you can all take:

- Live a Healthy Brain Lifestyle with appropriate diet, exercise, and following the Six Pillars of Brain Health.
- Promote awareness of the importance of early detection and evaluation of memory loss symptoms.
- Support organizations that promote the advancement of Alzheimer's research and treatment. Some recommendations:
  - National Alzheimer's Association alz.org
  - Alzheimer's Orange County (local) Alzoc.org
  - The HealthyBrainClub.com
  - Global Alzheimer's Platform Foundation globalalzplatform.org

You've finished. Before you go…

Tweet/share that you finished this book.

Please star rate this book.

Reviews are solid gold to writers. Please take a few minutes to give us some itty bitty feedback.

ABOUT THE AUTHOR

Dr. Trinh is Chief Medical Officer of Irvine Clinical Research, focused on Alzheimer's Research.

He is a well-known expert in speaking on memory loss and brain health. He has shared educational and medical knowledge on television, religious centers, local colleges, medical centers, senior centers, and at Alzheimer's Orange County, where he is a board member.

He is the President and Founder of HealthyBrainClub.com dedicated to promoting awareness and education about brain health.

He is the President and Founder of the PhysiciansCBDcouncil.com, dedicated to advocate for cannabis medical research for therapeutic opportunities.

If you enjoyed this book you might also like…

- **Your Amazing Itty Bitty® Heal Your Body Book** – Patricia Garza Pinto
- **Your Amazing Itty Bitty® Diet Free Weight Loss Book** – Liz Bull
- **Your Amazing Itty Bitty® Weight Loss Book** – Suzy Prudden and Joan Meijer-Hirschland

And many more Itty Bitty® books available on line.

www.ingramcontent.com/pod-product-compliance
Lightning Source LLC
Chambersburg PA
CBHW071752050426
42335CB00065B/1783